Low-Carb Coach

HAVE YOUR BACON AND EAT IT TOO

Jason Vriends

Contents

I dedicate this book to my wife, Deborah Vriends, who allowed me the freedom to try new things, make mistakes, learn, and grow. I couldn't have done it without you. I love you with all my heart.

We cannot solve our problems by using the same kind of thinking we used when we created them.

—ALBERT EINSTEIN

ACKNOWLEDGEMENTS

Thanks to the man I met one day on the bus in 2003, Mike Scott. It was your kindness that opened the door for me to walk through and allowed me to take charge of my life. Thank you for introducing me to this amazing meal plan and ultimately leading me to finally finding the cure to my food addiction and weight problem. I am truly grateful to have you as a friend.

Thanks to Peter Lalic. Without your experience in writing "The Book on Mobile Marketing", your knowledge, encouragement, and continually nudging me along, this book would not have been possible.

Thanks to Jerry and Debbie Papousek for introducing me to Nutrichem, which helped me conquer my anxiety and allowed me to finally break free of my plateau in order to reach a goal I never thought I could. Also, thanks for your friendly reminders that I don't need to eat like I used to, even though on Atkins I could have gotten away with it. Your ongoing encouragement and support helped me get through one of the most difficult times in my life.

I would like to extend my thanks to my editor Rebecca Mirzabozorg, who, being so knowledgeable about low-carb diets, provided valuable editing and input into this piece. Thank you for agreeing to take on this book and turning out such great work.

Thank you, Judi Maragh, for your ability in grammar and your critical thinking in writing. You really helped clarify the ideas in my head, allowing me to write them in this piece in an easy-to-understand way. Without your guidance, some of the information I wished to share with readers may have been lost in translation in my mind.

With the wealth of information that I have acquired through reading materials published by Gary Taubes, author of "Why We Get Fat"; Robert Atkins, author of "The Atkins Diet"; and Jimmy Moore, who wrote "Livin' La Vida Low-carb blog", I gained insight on how to effectively change my food habits, find alternative means to address my food allergies and sensitivities, and ultimately to create a long-term food plan that is easy to follow.

Finally, I would like to thank my parents, John and Karen; and brother, Cody, for putting up with my burping, hospital trips, doctor visits, and anxiety attacks which often kept you up late at night. You were patient and knew things would change for the better.

CHAPTER ONE

My Struggle

For most of my life, the dominant topic on my mind had been food. No matter where I was or what I was doing, my next food fix was always front and centre. Whether it was writing a test for school, working at a part-time job or even playing video games late at night, food was always my preoccupation.

Elementary school

During the period that I attended elementary school, I delivered newspapers, cut grass, raked leaves, and plowed snow to earn extra money--much of which was joyfully spent on food. Each weekend, my friends and I would rent Super Nintendo games from the local convenience store; buy chips, pop, candy and all the junk food under the sun; and settle in for the weekend. Our entire weekend comprised of playing video games and eating junk food.

This crucial period of my life basically set the assumption that this lifestyle was okay for me to have forever. It's easy to assume that certain aspects of our lives are okay simply because we don't see immediate consequences; however, the mere fact that I had set the habit of eating junk constantly became a very harsh consequence for a big chunk of my life.

High school

Throughout high school, the amount of food I ate for lunch would vary greatly. I'd either consume five whole plates of Chinese food at a local establishment called Ming's Restaurant, 20 Chicken McNuggets with an Apple Pie at McDonald's, or a measly Toonie Tuesday meal at KFC, which would land me two pieces of chicken and fries.

I also worked at Burger King for the few years I attended high school. During busy periods, burgers were made in advance so that customers would not have to wait. Each burger was marked with the time it was made, and after 10 minutes it was destined for the trash. Instead of throwing the food out, the manager allowed me to take it home, and I definitely couldn't say no to that offer. When orders of chicken nuggets came on the screen for 6 or 12, I would occasionally drop a few extra into the fryer so that I could nibble on them as I worked.

I also dressed up as a clown for Burger King Birthday parties just so I could get a piece of cake and candy. Once per week, the ice cream and milkshake machines were cleaned and, instead of throwing out the milkshake mix, I would fill up 32-ounce cups and bring them home. Being an employee has significant benefits for your average glutton, such as the 50% employee discount on purchases. As if that wasn't enough, on the days I wasn't working I would still buy food at Burger King, because it was more convenient than making it myself. I had quite literally become the king of burgers!

College

During the period that I attended college in New Brunswick, I worked at two jobs to supplement my student loan. To keep up the trend of free food, when I worked in the college cafeteria, the cook always gave me leftovers to take home. This meant that the cookies, muffins and sweets were mine by default as they were always baked in excess. Each week when it was time to clean the machine that was used for making "slushies", I would pour the contents into a jug and take it to my residence for a treat. Sadly, I didn't realize that it doesn't count as being a 'treat' if you regularly consume the goodies—it counts as a staple.

My second job was at a local convenience store, which provided me with sufficient funds to buy pizza pockets, treat bags, pop, and chips.

Living in residence at college was more of the same. In the evenings after eating the cookies, muffins, and sweets that I had taken home from the cafeteria, I would order a Big New Yorker from Pizza Hut. I always seemed to have a coupon for 10% off, so I typically ordered one of these every other night. In addition to that, I would purchase tubs of sour soothers and bubble gum from Costco, along with chips, cases of pop, and any other goodies I could find.

While playing computer games late into the night, I often paid people to drive me to Burger King, Wendy's, or the Salisbury

Irving Big Stop so I could get food because I felt so hungry. Eating loads of carbs makes you crave loads of carbs!

I remember one night, while I was watching TV in the lounge of my dorm, a girl walked in and asked if anyone would help her out, because her car wouldn't start. I decided to be the hero; hey, it was a girl after all! After helping her jumpstart her car, I ended up lying in a nearby snow bank for about thirty minutes to catch my breath. I believed it was certain that someone would have had to jumpstart my heart!

The Breaking Point

The breaking point came when I visited Jungle Jim's, a downtown restaurant in Moncton, New Brunswick. I ordered what's called the Kitchen Sink, because I thought I could consume it all. This meal was literally served in a stainless steel domestic sink. It came with Buffalo wings, monkey fingers, BBQ chicken taquitos, onion rings, lattice fries, garlic baguette, cauliflower, broccoli, carrots and celery sticks with blue cheese dressing and honey mustard dipping sauce.

I finished the meal with no problem and was rewarded with a high-five from my girlfriend (now my wife) along with an upset stomach and a lovely evening of vomiting. That was the final straw for my body, because from that point forward; I experienced bloating, gas, constant burping, acid reflux, anxiety, and a variety of minor nuisances. It had become so bad that in order to relieve the pressure from bloating and gas build-up, I had to force myself to burp. Doing this sometimes caused me to choke, and I became nervous of travelling anywhere without bottles of water.

I was so bloated that breathing was difficult, and simple exercise, such as climbing stairs, would cause me to have chest pains, sweating, heart palpitations, and I would often even think I was having a heart attack when it was simply gas. Each visit to the hospital would only yield test results showing anxiety or acid reflux. In order to resolve the bloating, anxiety, and gas problems, as well as the constant burping, while trying to keep the symptoms under control, I frequently had to visit doctors and specialists. I even had an endoscopy done, but nothing would help.

After college, the situation wasn't any better. I went back to Prince Edward Island (PEI) and began working at a call center. I used to take rolls of quarters with me to purchase candy from the two vending machines in the building. There were some delicious sour candies called "Chews" and soap-tasting gum called "Thrills" that I just could not get enough of.

I would often send out emails to co-workers to schedule runs to Dairy Queen. This gave me an excuse for a break and to have a Blizzard®. On other days, I would go to the local bakery and order a twelve-inch sub sandwich and a bag of chips. Sometimes I did both the Blizzard® and the foot-long!

Later on, I was hired to work for the federal public service, but it was located in Summerside, PEI. While working there, I never brought a lunch; the cafeteria had cinnamon rolls with a self-serve container of icing ready for me to scoop up, and I would have one or two of these during each break. For lunch, I would rotate between Wendy's and eating at the cafeteria, and there was very little difference between the two!

I always ate supper at home. For me, this was usually meat and potatoes or sloppy joes. My mom went to Bingo for a night out once or twice a week. When Mom did this, Dad and I would have a boy's night out, which consisted of watching movies and eating. Dad and I would make spaghetti with hamburger and tomato soup. After that meal I would eat boxes of cookies, bags of licorice, and whatever else I could find until I got sick and started throwing up.

Moved to Ottawa

In order to continue working in the public service, I needed to relocate to Ottawa and work at their headquarters. This was my first time far away from PEI, where the largest city I had lived in at the time had a population of a mere twenty thousand. At work, it was common for a team leader or manager to have candy at her or his desk for employees to nibble on from time-to-time. Instead of having a few, I would take a handful, often clearing out the dish whenever I would pass by.

On the way home from work, I was typically hungry before supper and would often visit the local Tim Horton's and purchase a dozen donuts. The walk from Tim Horton's to my house was five minutes, yet in this short period of time, I was able to devour between six to eight donuts, leaving only a few for my wife. After walking through the door and offering my wife the remainder of the donuts, she would always put them aside until after supper. That gave me extra time to have another one (or three). (I always tried to save her at least one donut, though.)

Having suffered with anxiety, bloating, chest pains and acid reflux for so long, I was used to the symptoms by this time, and
they no longer scared me. I decided to stop taking Paxil® and
Nexium® in order to figure things out for myself. I realized that
when I had burped enough, this often relieved the pressure in
my stomach and all the previously mentioned symptoms would
disappear. Unfortunately for those around me, I would need to
burp about every thirty seconds to keep up with the amount of
pressure I experienced in my stomach.

After a year in Ottawa, this ordeal wasn't any better, until one
day I was riding the bus with a friend. On that particular day,
my friend introduced me to a friend of theirs named Michael
Scott. As I inhaled five pieces of licorice at once, he apparently
noticed my weight and machine-like consumption of junk food
and felt the need to overwhelm me with information about the
Atkins Diet. After a few minutes, he realized that I wasn't really
interested in anything he had to say; and just to drive the point
home I ate even faster as he talked.

But then, every day as I rode the bus to and from work and
talked to Mike, I learned a little more and received the answers
to my questions. I said to myself, 'Here is a guy that is over sixty
years old and is in better shape than anyone I know. Who am I
going to listen to: my doctor, the news, or a man who has
proven results and an answer to each of my questions'?

Eventually I made a commitment to Mike that I would try going
low-carb for two weeks and that I would give it my best, which

I did. Wouldn't you know, I've been going strong for over ten years now!

For the first five years on the Atkins Diet, I lost weight but still had cravings every few weeks. I would ultimately crack and eat the naughty foods, in a machine-like fashion, which in turn made me gain more weight. As my weight-loss slowly continued, my discipline also increased to allow me to stick more to the low-carb foods. However, I still encountered burping, acid reflux, and several other digestion problems along with continued anxiety. To try and resolve these persistent problems, I saw doctors and specialists, took tests, and read articles online; in the end, nothing worked. I also spent hundreds of dollars on supplements, but none of those helped either. The anxiety became so bad that I would shake, sweat, and be scared of seemingly normal or day-to-day situations that happened all the time.

One day, a new employee at work started to notice and point out my constant burping and questioned me on it. This was the first time someone actually confronted me on the issue, and I was shocked. After describing my problem to the new employee (now friend), Jerry Papousek recommended I take my problems to Kent MacLeod, the owner of the Nutrichem Compounding Pharmacy. Nutrichem specializes in drug-free health solutions. I purchased their Body Chemistry Balancing (BCB) package, and they evaluated my digestion, hormone levels, antioxidants, energy production, neurotransmitter function, gastrointestinal health and general metabolism.

When the test results came back, I met with Kent MacLeod and discussed the results. After seeing the high cortisol levels in the blood work and hearing the description of my gas problems, I was told that my problems were likely due to food intolerances. To combat this problem, Kent suggested I try an elimination diet. I ended up removing dairy and eggs, wheat, soy and gluten, as well as taking probiotics and digestive enzymes. After 3 months, I started to see successful results from removing soy, dairy, eggs, and wheat from my diet; however, I still wasn't a hundred percent better. I logged my results as I ate certain foods, but started to become afraid of eating almost everything, as I feared almost every food would trigger my anxiety or gas problems.

I prayed to God that if I could be healed from this horrible problem, I would glorify Him in front of the entire congregation at our church and would start changing my ways. Returning to see Kent, we carried out another test called an IGG food test, which identifies specific foods to which a person may be intolerant. Kent found the test results almost overwhelming, with the number of items to which I reacted. Almost everything returned a reaction, from wheat, to eggs, dairy, soy, nuts, and so much more!

Instead of having to guess which foods were triggering my problems, I finally had something to go by. One-by-one, I started removing these foods from my diet and before I knew it, things became almost normal. Not only did my anxiety subside, I lost the extra weight, from 225 lbs. that I had plateaued at to now 180 lbs. To read more about my personal story or to see my before and after results, visit _lowcarbcoach.com_.

Kent made up a custom formula consisting of the vitamins and supplements that my body required (based on my blood work), and I avoided the foods that were identified as intolerances. All the doctors had suggested taking Paxil® for anxiety and Zantac® or Nexium® to control my digestive issues. No one took the time to determine the root cause of my symptoms (food intolerance). They just tried to push pills in a one-size-fits-all manner.

I kept my promise and announced my story to our church. I presented my knowledge on food intolerances, the low-carb lifestyle, and the theory on why we get fat to the entire congregation. Later, a friend named Peter Lalic, who recently wrote "The Book on Mobile Marketing", suggested that I share my knowledge in the same format that he did, and this book is the result. Aren't you lucky?

Since that first day over 10 years ago, Michael and I have remained friends, and because of his introduction to a low-carb diet, I have surpassed my original goal of 220 lbs. and have finally reached my new goal of 180 lbs. While most believe that you need to balance diet and exercise to be fit and healthy, I accomplished this all through a low-carb diet alone with absolutely no exercise! This isn't to say that you can't exercise if you so choose, in fact it's encouraged, but rather that it's entirely possible to *only* eat this way to fit back into your favorite jeans.

From holidays to birthdays, there will be an indulgence from time-to-time. However, with the right tools and right information that I have spent so much time figuring out, as well as the results that I have had thus far, I know that I can get right back on track and continue with a working plan; using the tools I'll provide you with, you will, too!

CHAPTER TWO

Low-Carb Explained

ow-carb diets limit the amount of foods you can eat which contain large amounts of carbohydrates; such as breads, cereals, pasta, fruits, starchy vegetables, milk products, as well as sugary foods; like candy, syrups, and jams. Instead of consuming high-carb foods, those following a low-carb diet eat meat, poultry, fish, shellfish, eggs, cheese, nuts and seeds. These people also eat low-carb vegetables and fruits, like green leafy salads, avocado, and berries.

What Happens When You Eat Carbs?

All carbohydrates, except for dietary fiber, are ultimately broken down into sugar. After eating too many carbs, your blood sugar rises and insulin is released to remove the extra carbohydrates from the blood stream and stores them in the fat cells. Insulin is a storage hormone which tells the body to store the extra carbs as fat and blocks the body from using stored fat as fuel. The extra carbs not only make you fat, they make sure you stay fat.

The longer sugar remains in your blood stream, the greater the risk of your body being damaged. Over time, sugar behaves like a slow-acting poison, causing complications such as kidney disease, strokes, heart-attacks, and poor circulation to the legs and feet. Eventually, you become insulin resistant and instead of only releasing the right amount of insulin to remove the excess carbs from your blood stream, your pancreas overreacts. It then releases too much insulin, and instead of removing just the right amount of sugar, it removes it all. This causes your blood sugar to become too low, causing cravings for more carbs. This is known as the Blood Sugar Rollercoaster.

This is the primary reason that type II diabetics have such acute health problems. After years of overcompensating, their pancreas becomes unable to produce enough insulin. This leads to high blood sugar for long periods of time, resulting in damage being caused to their bodies.

As long as you keep your insulin low, your body will use fat as its fuel source instead of glucose. This is the reason people lose weight so quickly on a low-carb diet and do not have the cravings associated with low-fat or low-calorie diets.

The primary culprit here is the sleeping glucagon; when you eat a lot of carbs, your body keeps producing insulin and keeps glucagon in a sort of coma. Once you're eating a sensible number of carbs through the aide of a low-carb diet, glucagon will "wake up" and start burning your fat for you. This is why high-carb dieters have such a hard time burning fat without excessive exercise, which is the only way for them to burn through the carbs and awaken the glucagon! Low-carb dieters don't have this issue because their body eats through the carbs rather quickly and goes straight to the glucagon; additionally, low-carb dieters who keep their carb levels to 50 net carbs or under go into a state of "ketosis", accelerating their weight loss. There's more information on this in the next two chapters, but if you have questions and want human contact, feel free to join our community at _lowcarbcoach.com_ and ask away to your heart's content!

Why Start a Low-carb Diet?

There are many benefits that come along with starting a low-carb diet. Several studies have concluded benefits such as: greater weight loss with a low-carb diet vs. low-fat/low-calorie diets, improved good cholesterol, decreased bad cholesterol, lower blood sugar, improved insulin sensitivity, decreased blood pressure and a lower blood insulin level, which is responsible for burning fat. High-carb diets can cause excess yeast to accumulate in your body, making a person feel mentally foggy or even contribute to anxiety and depression.

We have always been told that the answer to losing weight is simple: _eat less and exercise more._ If you have ever tried to limit your calories or reduce your fat intake, you will agree that it is very difficult, if not impossible, to sustain. With some willpower and support, you can do it for a while, but then you will eventually "go off the wagon" and return to your old ways. You may have lost some weight in the past, but eventually put it back on because you couldn't keep up the reduced caloric or fat intake for any length of time. Not to mention the fact that you need to adjust the amount of calories you eat every time you lose weight, constantly keeping yourself at the same hunger levels as your body shrinks.

Why can't you sustain reduction of your fat or caloric intake? It's because you're eating carbs! This causes you to crave more carbs; when you deliberately limit how much you eat, you soon feel hungry again. Anyone who has tried to eat less for a long time has discovered that it is very difficult. What you're eating is making you want to eat more, but you mentally make yourself eat less. Eating less than you want for the rest of your life is something almost anyone would find difficult at best.

On a low-carb diet, you can eat as much as you want, as long as the food is low in carbohydrates. You also don't have to count calories! What if I told you that you could eat foods such as steak, bacon, "breaded" fried chicken, buttery fried mushrooms and parmesan roasted vegetables, a variety of eggs and omelets, raspberries and strawberries with dark chocolate or whipped cream without *any* guilt, and that that's just the tip of the iceberg?

A low-carb diet means that your body will be using fat as its primary energy source instead of glucose. This makes it easier to lose weight and to keep it off--all this while not being the slightest bit hungry. The majority of people have a fairly difficult time dieting because of the diet's restrictive nature; we all know that not being able to eat as much as we want whittles away at our motivation until there's no motivation left. You wanted the "secret"; the key to success? Well, I'm giving it to you right here, and it's never been easier!

Benefits of Low-Carb Diets

When you choose a diet, you want to make sure there are plenty of positive benefits beyond losing weight. You want to be healthier overall by eating in the manner the diet instructs you to eat on a daily basis. You also want to be able to follow the plan for life instead of just a few weeks or months. The benefits of a low-carb diet will provide a healthy daily plan that you can implement for life.

You may not realize that eating a high amount of carbs can increase the chance of negative health issues. By reducing your carb intake, some medical conditions you have experienced in the past may occur less often. The frequency of headaches, joint pain, and trouble concentrating will usually diminish when you reduce your carb intake. This may help you reduce the amount of pain medicine you take because the pain of headaches and joints go away.

Often when you diet, mood swings can cause the process to be difficult. The highs and lows of your mood and energy can cause you to binge eat. Another benefit of the low-carb diet is the balancing of mood and energy. The body actually gets more consistent energy from protein and fat than from carbs, which may surprise you since athletes all load up on carbs before a game. This is because carbs bring on short-term energy spurts that will drop your energy level quickly once the carbs are gone. However, by reducing your carb intake, your energy will come from ketones. Ketones are basically the by-products of when your fatty acids are broken down; the result is a far more consistent source of energy that even your heart and brain use. This is why low-carb marathon runners don't hit a wall in the middle of a race—they actually gain energy!

If you enjoy exercise and want to tone and build muscle tissue, which helps fight fat in your body, a low-carb diet can help. After a workout, your muscles are very sensitive to insulin and do not need as many carbs as some people may think; instead, they should be fed protein to battle the upcoming soreness from your workout. By eating a low-carb diet, your muscles will draw in more amino acids from your meals after a workout; the amino acids will help the muscles heal from the workout faster and burn even more fat.

The impact or prevention of diabetes can be helped by a low-carb diet. If you have diabetes, a low-carb diet may help balance your insulin level throughout the day. If you have family members with diabetes and want to avoid getting the disease yourself, a low-carb diet is a good and healthy way to naturally balance your insulin.

Low-carb diets increase energy, reduce cravings for sweets-- sometimes completely--providing better mental concentration and greatly reducing or even eliminating "compulsive" or "emotional" eating. Also, dental checkups are greatly improved as a result of reduced sugar consumption, which the bacteria on your teeth love to chow down on.

You can also expect relief for joint or muscle pain, fewer headaches, reduced gastrointestinal symptoms (e.g. heart burn), and improved skin appearance.

As you can see, there are many benefits to a low-carb diet beyond just losing weight. You will see an improvement in your weight, but you will also have more energy and feel healthier. That is the goal of losing weight, as well: to be healthier overall, even though to look aesthetically pleasing is a bonus.

Are Low-Carb Diets Healthy?

According to our experts, we should "eat a balanced diet." What does this mean? Should we eat equal portions of fat, carbs, and protein? Should we make sure to eat something from all the food groups, like one part meat, one part potato, and one part milk? I don't know about you, but if it's going to make me fat, cause health problems, or give me diabetes, then it doesn't seem like a great idea to me.

We should be eating whatever is good for us. If that means cutting the bread, pasta, rice, and potatoes out of the diet and replacing it with meat and high-fiber fruits and veggies, then that likely is a balanced diet.

Public health authorities and institutions have been recommending low-fat and low-calorie diets for as long as I can remember. A lot of food companies making packaged products have a vested interest in such diet programs and have been promoting them for years. It is very difficult to admit being wrong, especially if recommendations have been made to so many people. If you hear something day in and out from your doctor, TV, and the radio, it's easy to become very convinced of what is being said; I believe some people like to call that "brainwashing".

There have been many studies about low-carb diets, and they are all positive. When on a low-carb diet, you can expect greater weight loss, improved good cholesterol, decreased bad cholesterol, lower blood sugar, improved insulin sensitivity, decreased blood pressure, lower blood insulin levels, and less muscle mass lost per pound.

One of the biggest myths about low-carb diets is that eating fat will give you heart disease. Several studies have shown that low-carb diets actually help to prevent heart disease. This information seems almost completely upside down to what we hear from our doctors, TV, and radio almost daily! Research is now vindicating Dr. Robert Atkins, who was promoting this point of view forty years ago.

Can Athletes Benefit from a Low-Carb Diet?

The first two things that come to mind when speaking to an athlete about a low-carb diet are that you need carbs for energy and that you lose muscle mass on a low-carb diet.

Study after study has concluded that as long as you're getting enough protein and fat while keeping your net carbohydrates (carbohydrates – fibers) below 20-30, you could lose a hundred pounds without losing muscle. It's true that your body needs carbs, but it actually doesn't need you to eat them! Your body will surprisingly convert fat into carbs, causing you to lose weight and allowing your body to have a constant energy source instead of variable energy. That is one of the reasons that carb-loading athletes often hit a wall midway through a race. They run out of carbs, and therefore energy. This is not a problem when you're on a constant energy source of your own personal fat. Additionally, it's been discovered by Dr. Atkins in his latest publication before his death, *Dr. Atkins' New Diet Revolution,* that if you are in lipolysis and eating low enough carbs to be in ketosis then your body will primarily burn fatty tissue, and therefore no lean body mass would be lost. Lipolysis is basically the fancy term for saying that your fat is being broken down and released into your body; since your body is focusing on breaking down your fat, then the weight you're losing is coming from the fat you're burning and not any sort of muscle loss!

The same is not true on a low-fat or low-calorie diet. On these diets, much of the weight loss is muscle, and that's not good, since muscle burns fat. Thus, losing your muscle would mean that you'll eventually lose fat a lot more slowly.

How Does a Low-Carb Diet Work?

Very low-carb diets limit the amount of carbs to between 20 and 30 carbohydrates per day, fibers not included. By reducing net carbs below 20 to 30 per day, the body will be guaranteed to enter into a state called ketosis (which is very different from ketoacidosis), which simply means that the body is burning fat for fuel instead of glucose.

However, many people can enter ketosis with a carb count of 50 per day, too, or even more. As everyone's body is different, the best way to determine what your carb intake level should be is to start at 20 net carbs until you're fully immersed in ketosis (this will usually take 3-4 days up to ten days). From there, if you are simply looking for your ketosis carb level then increase your carbs by 5 net carbs per week. Make sure to test yourself to see if you're in ketosis every few days using Ketostix or some other measure; if using Ketostix, then ensure that you're testing at the same time each time and that it isn't first thing in the morning as your urine will be concentrated at that point and will most likely return positive on the test strip regardless of whether or not you're in ketosis. Once you've reached a carb level where you're no longer in ketosis, decrease your net carbs by 5 and that should be your carbohydrate intake level to stay in ketosis! Keep in mind that on the days that you exercise, you will be able to eat a higher number of carbs and still be in ketosis.

While in ketosis, the body generates a minimal amount of insulin, so the body burns any fat that is eaten as fuel; if more is needed, then the fat cells freely release fat into the blood stream to be burned as fuel.

The difference between ketosis and ketoacidosis is that ketosis is simply when your body has an elevated level of ketone bodies whereas ketoacidosis is when your body can no longer regulate ketone production and accumulates keto acids, decreasing the pH of your blood and potentially being fatal. People oftentimes confuse the two because their names are so similar. You can tell when you're in ketosis when you're experiencing a lack of cravings, potentially have different-smelling urine through getting rid of excess ketones and possibly even have a foamy substance on top of your urine—you can test and confirm using Ketostix found at your local pharmacy or even using a blood ketone meter. Ketoacidosis is *only* a risk if you're diabetic or suffer from alcoholism, which isn't to say that low-carb diets won't or can't work for you, but rather that you should consult your physician to ensure that it's deemed safe.

Unlike the Blood Sugar Rollercoaster caused by carbohydrates, protein and fat satisfy your hunger. When you eat protein, you don't crave more protein. If you had a large plate of chicken, you would no longer continue to be hungry after you had had enough. You would eat a certain amount, and then you wouldn't need to eat anymore. You don't require a cheering section to keep you on your diet. After you finish your meal, you would be satisfied rather than craving more due to emotional eating. Even if you did want a bit of a "finale" to let your mind, rather than your stomach, know that your meal was finished, you could finish it off with a low-carb sweet, such as low-carb chocolate mousse, which is much richer in flavor than the low-calorie version due to the usage of real and natural ingredients!

Limiting yourself to 20-30 grams of carbs per day is still easier than reducing your calories on a low-fat or low-calorie diet. After a while, your cravings for carbohydrates will be greatly reduced. As your fat cells steadily release their fuel to be burned, instead of getting more difficult over time, eating low-carb actually becomes easier as your cravings subside.

Let's Recap

1. All carbs, except dietary fiber, are broken down into sugar in the body.

2. The body will not burn fat for fuel as long as there is a steady supply of sugar. Without sugar, the body will be forced to burn fat for energy.

3. The breakdown of fat will produce energy in the form of ketones for the body.

4. Insulin levels become stabilized when the pancreas no longer has to pump out large amounts in response to sugary, starchy meals or snacks.

5. By burning fat as fuel, you are no longer making and storing body fat, or having cravings, or blood sugar swings.

Low-carb diets will burn fat and preserve lean muscle. If you exercise, you will even add lean muscle while losing fat. Muscle weighs more than fat but takes up less bulk, so you may find yourself getting smaller in size without seeing a drastic drop on the scales. If you want to lose weight quickly and keep it off and actually improve your blood pressure, cholesterol, and overall health, a low-carb diet is the way to go.

Now that you understand low-carb diets, their benefits, and how they work, it's time to update what you thought you knew and help you understand that low-carb diets are safe, effective, and becoming more popular than ever.

CHAPTER THREE

Popular Low-Carb Diets

ooking through the bookstore can quickly cause you to become confused as to which popular low-carb diet to choose. Quite a few different authors have written books about low-carb diets, and they all have different ideas about the best way to go about it. In this chapter, I will describe the most popular low-carb diets, the basics of each diet, and the one that I selected for myself.

The Atkins Diet:

The Atkins Diet is also referred to as The Atkins Nutritional Approach. This low-carbohydrate diet was introduced by Robert Atkins. He had been inspired by a research paper entitled "Weight Reduction" by Dr. Alfred W. Pennington. Atkins used the concept to resolve his own problem of obesity.

The Atkins Diet is called The Atkins Nutritional Approach (ANA) as it provides health benefits; this explains the reason why many people should choose this nutritional approach regardless of whether or not they need to lose weight. Quality of life is just as important as being in a healthy weight range, and what's better than being energetic first thing in the morning while having decreased or totally eliminated any internal issues you may have had, within reason!

ANA is a lifetime eating plan. Dieters have to keep track of the quantity and quality of carbohydrates they consume, determine their personal carbohydrate threshold, and take mineral and vitamin supplements, and exercise. This isn't to say that you have to be a hardcore weight-lifter or even constantly do high intensity training, though these exercises would definitely complement your new eating lifestyle, but rather that you should ensure that you at least get to walk your dog around the block a few times or something equivalent. Pets have got to live a little, too!

This diet is customized to suit a person's metabolism. The ANA requires you to learn your threshold for carbohydrate consumption and reach your ideal goal weight. ANA can be called a program that helps you achieve permanent weight control through a reduced consumption of carbohydrates.

ANA follows four principles which include weight loss, weight maintenance, good health, and disease prevention.

The diet itself follows four phases:

Phase 1: Induction
Phase 2: Ongoing Weight Loss (OWL)

Phase 3: Pre-Maintenance
Phase 4: Lifetime Maintenance.

The transition from one phase to another allows you to achieve and maintain the right weight, develop good eating habits, feel good and reduce the risk of serious chronic diseases (e.g. heart disease, hypertension, or diabetes).

People can avoid the induction phase and move directly onto ongoing weight loss if they do not need to lose too much weight (< 15 pounds).

By studying the four principles of the Atkins Diet, you can learn more about the results you can expect.

Weight loss: The Atkins Diet helps both men and women shed weight quickly. In the event that your metabolism does not allow you to lose weight, there are means of overcoming such barriers.

Weight maintenance: Atkins Dieters do not complain of hunger pains as they discover their own effective level of carbohydrate intake.

Good health: Atkins encourages you to eat wholesome healthy food rather than junk food. When you learn to stabilize your blood sugar, you won't feel any fatigue or cravings.

Disease prevention: The carbohydrate-controlled diet results in lower insulin production--a blessing for people suffering from hypertension, diabetes, and cardiovascular disease.

Phase 1 - Induction

The first phase is the most restrictive but results in the fastest weight loss. This phase works based on a process called ketosis, which we mentioned earlier, but let's remind ourselves of what it is while learning a few new fun facts. While in ketosis, your body will burn fat for energy instead of carbs. It's recommended that you stay on this phase for at least two weeks, but may continue as long as required. For most people who are asked the question, "Do you want to lose weight faster or slower?" I am sure that the answer is faster. Well, if that's the case for you, then induction is your friend and you can stay on it until you're within reach of your weight loss goal (ideally within 15 pounds).

The Atkins Diet is not a low-calorie diet. Just because you're not eating carbs doesn't mean you are not eating. You should be eating as much protein as you need in order to be full while also eating sufficient amounts of fat. If you start reducing your calorie intake, your body may burn muscle instead of fat! Women should eat a minimum of 1500-1800 calories per day while men should be eating a minimum of 1800-2000 calories—as you can see, this is miles away from a low-calorie diet!

During the Induction phase, you need to limit carbohydrate consumption to 20 grams per day, not including fibers. You need to eat protein and fat-rich foods, such as fish, chicken, eggs, lamb, pork or beef, cheese; and get your carbohydrates from nutrient-dense foods, such as spinach. It's also important to drink a minimum of eight glasses of water per day, as low-carb diets act as a diuretic. However, like any other diet, please consult a physician before starting.

This diet works on the idea that if your body does not have carbohydrates to burn, it will burn fats instead.

Phase 2 - Ongoing Weight Loss (OWL)

At this point, your rate of weight loss will be slowing down. In the first week, you can increase your daily carb intake from 20 to 25 grams; the next week you move on to 30 grams. These 5 gram increments should be continued until your weight loss slows down to one or two pounds per week.

During this phase, you can start adding more nutrient-dense foods, such as broccoli, raspberries, nuts, seeds, and soft cheeses, but take note of which foods make your weight loss stall! This phase continues until you have roughly 10 pounds to lose until you reach your ideal goal weight.

Phase 3 - Pre-maintenance:

You need to lose the next few pounds slowly and maintain the desired weight for a month. You can slowly add lentils, legumes, other fruits, starchy vegetables, and whole grains. The desired goal weight is called the Atkins Carbohydrate Equilibrium, where your weight can either go up or down.

Phase 4 - Lifetime maintenance:

In this phase, the average number of daily grams of net carbs increases up to 120 grams per day. This depends on several factors, such as: gender, activity level, age, and metabolism. At this final phase, you feel good and move from diet to healthy lifestyle.

The South Beach Diet

The South Beach Diet is attributed to a cardiologist dietician duo: Arthur Agatston and Marie Almon. This diet is an alternative to low-fat diets, such as the Ornish Diet and Pritikin Diet, and was first developed as prevention for heart disease. The diet works on replacing the bad carbs and fats by good carbs and fats.

This diet is based on the fact that hunger cycles are triggered by carbohydrate-rich foods which the body takes no time in digesting; leading to a spike in blood sugar.

The South Beach Diet replaces bad carbohydrates with carbohydrates from unprocessed foods, like vegetables, beans, and whole grains. Carbohydrates are considered good if they have low glycemic index.

This diet eliminates trans-fats and discourages saturated fats, which are replaced with foods rich in unsaturated fats and Omega-3 fatty acids. The diet replaces fatty portions of red meat and poultry with lean meats, nuts and oily fish.

The South Beach Diet has three phases: the first phase lasts two weeks and its premise is to avoid fruits, grains, starches, and alcohol. The second phase depends on the dieter's desire for the amount of weight they want to lose. In this stage, some fruits, vegetables and grains are reintroduced. The third phase consists of the maintenance phase, which is meant to last a lifetime.

According to Agatston, the diet replaces bad fats and carbs by good ones and does not allow dieters to forego carbohydrates entirely.

The Zone Diet

This diet was introduced by the biochemist Barry Sears. It underlines the consumption of carbohydrates, proteins and fats in a balanced ratio – 40:30:30. Sears refers to a proper hormone balance as "The Zone". When the insulin levels are neither high nor low and glucagon levels are not too high, specific anti-inflammatory chemicals, eicosanoids, are released. The eicosanoids have the same effects as aspirin without the downsides of gastric bleeding. According to Sears, the 30:40 ratio of protein to carbohydrate triggers this effect named "The Zone". Under caloric balance, the human body fat is unable to store excess calorie as fat and burn it at the same time. The Zone also advocates a high Omega-3 to Omega-6 ratio.

Sears believes that a high proportion of carbohydrates compared to protein in a diet increases the production of insulin, which is responsible for the body storing more fat. Sears suggests that fat consumption is important for burning fat. Monounsaturated fats make a person feel full and decrease the rate at which carbohydrates are absorbed in the bloodstream. Slower carbohydrate consumption means lower insulin levels, which result in less stored fats and a faster transition to fat-burning. A person tends to feel fatigued if the body needs energy but is unable to burn fat due to high insulin levels. The brain feels starved and the metabolism is unable to compensate. This is because the brain functions on glucose but the high insulin level reduces the glucose level. This condition is referred to as rebound hypoglycemia.

Sears recommends that you eat protein as much as the palm of your hand, as much non-starchy raw vegetables as possible, enough carbohydrates to maintain mental clarity, and enough monounsaturated oils to keep hunger away.

The Paleo Diet

The Paleo Diet is known by several other names: Caveman diet, Stone Age diet, Primal diet, and Hunter Gatherer diet, to name a few. This modern diet considers a diet of wild plants and animals consumed by hominid species in the Paleolithic era. This diet is attributed to a gastroenterologist Walter L. Voegtlin. It is based on the assumption that modern humans are genetically adapted to the diet of their Paleolithic ancestors and that human genetics has not changed since then.

The diet revolves around foods that are available in the present, such as fish, grass-fed pasture-raised meats, eggs, vegetables, fruit, fungi, roots, and nuts. It excludes grains, legumes, potatoes, dairy products, refined sugar, and processed oils. Oils with low Omega-6 to Omega-3 ratio, like olive oil or canola, are allowed. Dieters can have water and tea, but must avoid alcoholic and fermented beverages. Contrary to what you might think, food in this diet should be cooked, although some raw Paleo Dieters stick to uncooked food.

The GI Diet:

Glycemic Index (GI) ranks carbohydrates based on their quality and their ability to raise blood sugar levels after a meal. The index has a scale of 1 to 100 of foods in order of release of sugar on consumption.

Carbohydrates are divided into three categories:

1. High Glycemic Index foods (GI 70 and above) lead to an immediate rise in blood sugar.

2. Intermediate Glycemic Index foods (GI 55-69) cause an average rise in blood sugar.

3. Low Glycemic index foods (GI 55 or below) induce slow release of blood sugar.

High value GI foods increase the level of sugar in our blood, induce hunger pains and lead to excessive food intake and obesity. Low GI foods, on the other hand, produce low blood sugar levels, regulate hunger pains and prevent unnecessary food intake. Low GI foods help people avoid obesity and cardiovascular disease.

Oats, oat bran, fruit, and toasted muesli with milk are a good way to start your day. Oats have low GI and can be added to milkshakes. Grilled fish and meat with vegetables are also low in GI. Include one low GI meal in your diet. Nuts (e.g. almonds, walnuts, cashews, peanuts) and frozen, low-fat fruit desserts are low in GI. Eat fruits like apples, cherries, plums, pears, peaches, grapes, oranges, strawberries, prunes, kiwi and vegetables like cauliflower, cabbage, tomatoes, lettuce, chilies, and onions.

The Sugar Buster Diet

This diet advises dieters to cut down on sugar to get rid of their fat. The Sugar Buster Diet was introduced by four authors: Leighton Steward, a former CEO; Dr. Morrison C. Bethea, a cardiothoracic surgeon; Dr. Samuel S. Andrews, an endocrinologist; and Dr. Luis A. Balart, a gastroenterologist.

According to this diet, you are supposed to eliminate refined sugar completely, as well as fruits and vegetables, which have high sugar content. With this diet, you can control your cholesterol, obtain a feeling of well-being, increase your energy, and treat your diabetes and other diseases.

The diet bans certain foods, like potatoes, corn, refined sugar, corn syrup, molasses, honey, sugared colas, and beer. You can have high-fiber vegetables, stone-ground whole grains, lean and trimmed meats, fish and some fruits. Use oil high in mono- and poly-unsaturated fats and low in saturated fats.

Let's Recap

1. The Atkins Diet propagates low-carb diets for metabolic advantage because burning fat takes more calories, so you expend more calories. According to this theory, hunger is the reason that low-fat diets fail and the Atkins Diet provides adequate protein, fat, and fiber to prevent hunger.

2. Agatston came out with the South Beach Diet as he feared that the Atkins Diet would lead to too little carbohydrates and fiber and too much saturated fats, which could lead to a risk of heart disease. This theory suggests replacing bad carbs and fats with good ones.

3. The Zone Diet by Sears proposes a diet of carbohydrates, protein, and fats in a balanced ratio. According to Sears, low-carb diets ignore the importance of moderation and balance. The Zone Diet espouses a moderate carb diet.

4. The Paleo Diet proclaims that 56-65% of food energy should be derived from meat and 36-45% from plant sources. The propagators of this diet mention that excessive consumption of foods, like refined vegetable oils, refined sugars, dairy products, cereals and alcohol can lead to obesity, cardiovascular disease, high blood pressure, osteoporosis, type II diabetes, and cancer.

5. The GI Diet recommends low GI index foods. This diet has been criticized because foods have certain factors that contribute to the food's glycemic level, such as ripeness, food processing, cooking method and plant variety.

Why I chose the Atkins Diet

After researching the various diet plans, I selected the Atkins Nutritional Approach for my personal weight loss and ongoing maintenance. Unlike other weight-loss programs, Atkins provides phases, so it can be individualized. This phased approach enabled me to burn the amount of fat I wished while controlling my weight loss based on my ongoing needs. For example, if one week I wanted a bit more carbs as a treat, I could move into a higher phase and then move back into Induction when I wanted to speed up my weight loss again.

Almost 10 years later, I still consider myself to be in the Induction phase; I found that when I increased my carbs, my cravings for more carbs also increased. This is again a great tool, as you can adjust your phase based on the cravings, desired weight loss speed, and personal factors.

Having a system that allows me to move between various levels of carbohydrate intake based on my needs during that particular week is an essential asset. I know that if at any time I start to gain weight from the higher phases, I can always move down to a lower phase where the carbs are more restrictive. This is great for people with diabetes, as they may end up staying on the Induction phase for the rest of their lives. The good news is that regardless of what phase you're in, you still won't be hungry and will not have cravings.

The other diet or weight loss programs jump out, making you feel warm and fuzzy, as they allow "natural" sugar or "good carbs". Some even limit the amount of saturated fat, which makes it more acceptable for traditional nutritionists and medical professionals. The issue with this is simple: the majority of people are insulin-resistant, and even "natural" sugar or "good carbs" are enough to start the Blood Sugar Rollercoaster. This isn't to say that you can't have sweets ever again—there are plenty of substitutes which are also natural but free of carbs! We'll discuss this more in the Getting Started chapter, or check out *lowcarbcoach.com* for some ideas.

People often attribute cravings to lack of willpower, but the truth is that cravings have biochemical origins. Blood sugar imbalances cause powerful cravings and this leads people to spend their days on a rollercoaster of blood sugar highs and lows, constantly eating to correct the imbalances.

You will find that the more healthy saturated fats you eat, the fuller you will feel. Fats such as butter, olive oil, and coconut oil are essential to being successful on a low-carb diet. In fact, there are even some tasty treats you can make that are almost entirely made up of fat—it may sound scary at first, but if you stop to consider the practically poisonous foods you're putting in your body as it is and try to scavenge for hard evidence as to why fatty foods is bad, you'll realize that it isn't so bad after all.

Robert Atkins really emphasized that you can eat as much as you wanted on the Atkins Diet, provided that the food you were eating was low in carbohydrates. As a food addict, these words were all I needed. I was so scared to start a low-carb diet at first, as all of the previous diets that I had tried or read about limited the quantity of food; it was practically like you felt starving or deprived constantly!

Robert Atkins used the ploy "eat as much as you want" because when people think about giving up carbs, it is hard to imagine, so it provides some compensation. But what people don't realize is that once you're past the first few days and your carb cravings have subsided, your desire to consume "as much as you want" goes down. You'll be eating more than you did before,

but you won't feel the need to overindulge yourself by any
means.

CHAPTER FOUR

Getting Started

ost people have been cutting their fat and reducing their calories for so long that they simply can't imagine increasing their intake of saturated fats or following a low-carb diet.

Initially, you may still crave carbs while your body converts from burning carbs to ketosis (burning fat). After a few days of low-carb eating, your blood sugar will stabilize, insulin levels will be greatly reduced, and your weight and cravings for carbohydrates will start dropping.

Every once in a while, you may miss carbs, but as you get used to this new way of eating, you'll think about it less and less. You will be content, satisfied, and never hungry, and not nearly as obsessed with food as you used to be.

My choice between always being hungry on low-calorie or low-fat diets versus never being hungry on a low-carb diet was an easy one for me.

Preparation

Before starting a low-carb diet, you need to be prepared. Being prepared includes everything from shopping, clearing out the junk food from your pantry, knowing what to eat and what to avoid, and documenting your vital signs.

Almost everyone regrets not taking measurements and/or pictures before starting a low-carb diet, so please take this step. Having your "before" weight, measurements, blood pressure, blood lipids, and blood glucose ensures that you can compare your success outside of just the scales.

Ideally, you will document your measurements and blood work every 6 to 12 months so you can have something to compare against. The reason for this is to be able to compare your success with your cholesterol numbers, say, six months from your start date, in order to see how far you've come. You could even take note of smaller successes, say, once every month.

Once you start losing weight, several of your friends may start making comments such as, "But I bet your blood pressure or cholesterol level is high". Having these numbers will allow you to demonstrate your success not just visually to your friends but also scientifically.

These are the things you should document:

Weight: You should weigh yourself on a scale that you'll have easy access to, and remember to weigh yourself at the same time of each day. Generally most people choose to weigh themselves each morning before breakfast, as your weight won't be influenced by water weight or any other factors at that point.

Body Fat Percentage: Generally, we talk about losing weight, but our ultimate goal is to lose fat. Many of the new scales today will provide you with this number, though if you'd like a more accurate result, then skin fold calipers are more accurate while DEXA scans or hydrostatic weighing are the most accurate—though they are rather expensive. An inexpensive way to check your body fat percentage is to simply use a tape measure and plug in the numbers into a body fat percentage calculator online.

Waist and Hip: Of greater importance than overall fat is something called "visceral fat" or "abdominal fat"; this is the fat that is around the organs and in our liver. You should measure your hips and waist, because some weeks you may not be losing fat but instead be losing inches off your waist and hips.

Blood Pressure: Blood pressure often responds well to a low-carb diet. If your blood pressure is high, you might want to track your blood pressure at home. If you are taking blood pressure medication, be sure to tell your doctor about your diet, as it's very common to need to change the amount of medication you will need. This is very important!

Blood Glucose: Your blood glucose after eating will be lower if you are eating fewer carbohydrates. Whether you are diabetic or not, you will want to measure this. If you are taking any medication for blood sugar, inform your doctor about the change in your diet.

<u>Blood Lipids:</u> Expect to see HDL, or "good" cholesterol, go up and LDL, or "bad" cholesterol, go down.

Shopping Advice

No special low-carb foods are needed. You can find nearly everything at a supermarket or grocery store in the meat, cheese, dairy and produce departments, or at your local farmer's market.

Watching carbs to lose weight or stay healthy should not cost you a fortune, which is why including high-priced foods in your diet is not necessary. There are countless less costly, yet delicious, options that are low in carbs. So let's get started on saving you money on the most delicious, low-carb foods!

We all know that packaged food is costly. Begin with home-cooked meals with dishes consisting of tender meat and fresh vegetables. Pre-packaged junk foods will only shrink your wallet in exchange for growing your waistline.

You may want to consider purchasing foods that are in season, like fruits and veggies when they are in season as they will taste better and will be cheaper. When produce is flown in from other countries, it is usually more expensive. By purchasing vegetables in season you can freeze them, allowing you to have your favorites all year around for less!

It's even possible to spend less on meat. While the expensive beef tenderloin is a tasty cut of meat, the chuck and sirloin cuts are also delicious meals at a much reduced price. They contain streaks of fat running throughout the meat, a thing that makes them tender, juicier and super delicious. They are best suitable to slow-cooking, as well as soups, stews, braises, and roasts.

In the same respect, protein that is priced right helps stretch your dollar, as well. Try looking for sales on meats and freezing them. There is more to controlling carbs than meat. Break the repetition of your dinner meat by including some eggs. Besides, you can prepare them in any way you like: poached, scrambled, omelet, or no-crust quiche, the options are limitless! Additionally, if you plan menus for your low-carb meals and know what you're going to eat ahead of time, then you can shop once a week or even once a month, freezing leftovers where appropriate. This will help with those pesky impulse purchases in addition to ensuring that you only have foods that you've planned for in advance!

You can save on snacks, too. Get low-carb snacks, including shakes and nutrition bars, for a cheap price during store specials. Try to buy these in bulk. Understand websites that offer items that you regard as your favorites, and sign up for their newsletters to catch their sales. Don't fail to check for coupons in newspaper circulars, as well.

Furthermore, make dishes that can serve as double recipes, so you can have dinner for one or two other nights. Likewise, make meals that can serve double-duty, like lunch the next day. Use your low-carb leftovers to stretch your dollar.

By planning your recipes and meals for the week, you can save time, money, along with willpower to not give in to urges for your old habits, too!

I recommend clearing your pantry of all unhealthy temptations, if you can: chips, candy, ice cream, sodas, juices, breads, and cereals. If you have other people living in your household who also consume these goods, perhaps consider having a locked pantry so you cannot access these naughty goods until you're either deep enough in ketosis to not be tempted or have enough willpower to say no.

Fibre Doesn't Count

By the way, when you're looking at labels to find out how many carbs something has, don't forget to subtract the fiber. "Net Carbs" are the total carbs minus the fiber. Fiber doesn't count. It is a carb, but you can't digest it. That's what fiber means: an indigestible carb. So, it doesn't have any effect on your insulin. It doesn't put sugar into your bloodstream; it just passes right through you.

For example, a stalk of broccoli has 8 grams of carbs; but 5 grams are fibers. So, a stalk of broccoli really has only 3 grams of carbs. That's what some labels call "net carbs" or "effective carbs."

What to Eat

This is merely a shortlist to get you started. You will find much more inspiration on the many low-carb websites, blogs, and books listed in the resources section.

When buying foods, always read the labels and always buy full-fat products. Never buy the low-fat, reduced fat or even zero-fat products. These products contain added sugar to replace the flavor removed when the fat was removed. Also, be sure to check the labels of products such as bacon, beef jerky, soup stocks, and deli meats as they often contain added sugar, fillers, or nitrates.

Below I've included a list of grocery items you can rotate through as a low-carb dieter.

Fats & Oils

- Butter
- Extra Virgin Coconut oil
- Fresh lard from naturally raised animals
- Extra Virgin, cold pressed, unfiltered Olive Oil
- Cold pressed nut oils for salad dressings
- Coconut milk

Protein

- Any and all cuts of Beef
- Any and all cuts of Pork
- Any and all cuts of Poultry
- Any and all cuts of Lamb or mutton
- Organ meats
- Fresh Eggs from poultry
- Fish and Shellfish

Cheese & Dairy

- Most cheeses, such as: triple cream brie, white cheddar, jarlsberg, gouda, parmesan, Monterey, mozzarella, stilton, or Havarti
- Cream cheese, full fat ricotta, or cottage cheese
- Cultured yogurt
- Heavy cream
- Half and half
- Sour cream

Canned Protein

- Sardines, herring, mackerel in water or olive oil
- Tuna and wild salmon in water
- Chicken, turkey, and beef
- Smoked herring
- Clams & oysters

Preserved Protein

- Sausages and bacon
- Beef Jerky – *watch out for added sugar*
- Pemmican, pork rinds
- Pickled eggs, herring

Vegetables

- Dark, leafy greens, such as kale, mustard greens, collards and chard
- Salad greens like romaine, iceberg, and spinach
- Summer squash, such as zucchini, crookneck, and patty pan

- Peppers, like green and red chilies
- Alliums like red and yellow onions, scallions, shallots, and garlic
- Broccoli, cauliflower, Brussels sprout
- Green beans, snow peas (not sweet peas)
- Green and red cabbage, Napa cabbage, endive, escarole
- Celery, cardoon, artichokes
- Eggplant, asparagus, cucumbers
- Turnips, kohlrabi, rutabaga
- Mushrooms, fresh or dried
- Fresh herbs
- Seaweed

Fruits

- Avocado & coconut
- Blueberries, blackberries, strawberries
- Cantaloupe & red grapes (these are higher in carbohydrates, so watch how many you eat)
- Canned organic tomatoes, tomato sauce, tomato paste

Frozen Foods

- Green beans, spinach, broccoli, cauliflower
- Whole cranberries, blueberries
- Meats, poultry and fish

Nuts and Seeds

- Raw almonds, pecans, walnuts, cashews
- Dry roasted almonds and macadamia nuts

- Hazelnuts and Brazil nuts
- Raw sunflower seeds, pumpkin seeds

Condiments & Spices

- Pickles
- Black and green olives
- Green or red salsa
- Canned green chilies
- Sauerkraut
- Taco enchilada sauce
- Horseradish and wasabi powder
- Tamari sauce and miso
- Fish sauce and toasted sesame oil
- Olive oil mayonnaise
- Clam juice, fish broth, chicken broth, and beef broth
- Pure vanilla
- All the herbs and spices your heart desires

What to Avoid

"Few people have 'old age' as a cause of death on their death certificate. Today we die of cancer, heart attacks, strokes, osteoporosis, diabetes, and so on. And we accept these conditions as normal causes of death. They aren't – and neither are ill-health, pain and discomfort that make our later years a misery.

"Do you practice 'healthy eating', consuming your 'five portions of fruit and vegetables' per day and shunning fats in favor of complex carbohydrates? Then you could be doing exactly what is most harmful to your health and helping to support one of the world's biggest most lucrative industries – the healthcare industry."

- Barry Groves, author of *Trick and Treat: How 'Healthy Eating' is making Us Ill.*

Below are the following things you should avoid and the reasons why.

Industrial Vegetable/Seed Oils

- Damages cell membranes
- Are too high in Omega-6 fatty acids
- Suppresses the immune system
- Can cause cells to become cancerous
- A major cause of macular degeneration

Industrial vegetable/seed oils include: canola, corn, soybean, "vegetable", peanut, sunflower, safflower, cottonseed, grape seed, and margarine.

Did you know - The fat content of the human body is about 97% saturated and monounsaturated fat, with only 3% polyunsaturated fats. Half of that three percent is Omega-3 fats, and that balance needs to be there. These oils contain very high levels of polyunsaturated fats, and these oils have replaced many of the saturated fats in our diets since the low-fat craze.

High Fructose Corn Syrup

- Fructose is a major contributor to insulin resistance
- Must be metabolized by the liver
- Contributes to non-alcoholic Fatty Liver Disease
- Causes a rise in serum glucose
- Zero nutrition

Grains and Brans

- Complex carbs are still carbs – *they are broken down into glucose*
- High in carbohydrates
- Low in nutrition
- Gluten is a cause of many gastrointestinal disorders
- Bran damages the lining of the intestine and colon

Processed Foods

- Not natural
- Contain many additives and preservatives
- Almost always contain added sugars and fake fats
- Made with the cheapest ingredients possible
- Low nutrition

High Sugar Fruits and Juices

- Contain fructose
- Cause a spike in serum glucose
- Cause a rise in serum insulin
- Relatively low in nutrition

Starchy Vegetables

- Complex carbs are still carbs – *they are broken down into glucose*
- Cause a rise in serum glucose
- Cause a rise in serum insulin

- May include if carbs are kept within a maximum limit per meal

Non-Fat and Low-Fat Dairy

- Contain too many carbohydrates
- Contain bad fats and synthetic ingredients

Unfermented Soy

- Physic acid inhibits absorption of minerals in the gut
- Phytoestrogens and isoflavones are toxic to estrogen sensitive tissues
- Protease inhibitors block the enzymes needed for protein digestion
- Goitrogens inhibit thyroid activity
- Exhibit carcinogenic effects

Additives and Preservatives

- Sodium benzoate
- Casein
- Sodium nitrate and nitrite

Manufactured protein sources

- Soy isolate (although this does lower bad cholesterol)

Sweeteners

- Agave syrup, Honey – *high in fructose*
- Maple syrup – raises blood glucose and insulin
- Splenda (increases insulin production by 20%), Sugar Twin, NutraSweet, Aspartame
- Sucrose
- Corn syrup
- Sugar alcohols – erythritol, maltitol, those ending in –ol (however, etythritol and xylitol don't seem to stall certain people, so if it works for you then go for it!)

Electrolytes

Traditional low-fat or low-calorie diets cause the body to store water. If you are following one of these diets, the addition of salt will cause your kidneys to store even more water, putting you at risk to have high blood pressure.

On a low-carb diet, your blood sugar will start to stabilize after 3-4 days, and your kidneys will begin to release all this extra fluid, and you will no longer store this extra water. While it's great to get rid of the excess toxins from our body more quickly, it comes at a cost. As the excess fluid leaves, it takes with it sodium and potassium. This can cause fatigue, headaches, light-headedness, dizziness, and cramping. If you are experiencing these symptoms, you have an imbalance of electrolytes.

Sodium: Ensure that you are adding sea salt to each of your meals. Since your blood sugar levels will stabilize, you will not be retaining the extra water and no, you will not get high blood pressure from the salt.

Potassium: Supplements can be purchased in 99-100mg dosages from your local pharmacy. I suggest taking between 2-4 tablets per day. **If you're on blood pressure medication, ask your doctor if it's okay to take potassium.**

Magnesium: Low-carb diets don't cause massive depletions of magnesium like it does with the sodium and potassium. However, most people who are overweight, insulin resistant, hypertensive or diabetic are deficient in magnesium. Magnesium Gluconate supplements can be purchased in 200mg dosages from your local pharmacy. I suggest taking 1-2 tablets per day. Magnesium is relaxing, so taking it in the evening will help you sleep and will also help you with constipation.

Food Substitutions

The most commonly asked question is probably: What about the comfort foods? You know, our favorites, like bread, rice, grains, and mashed potatoes. Try using some of the ideas below in place of your usual comfort foods for your next meal.

High-carb	Low-carb
Sugar	Stevia or Sucralose
Milk	Coconut, almond, or hemp milk (unsweetened)
Potatoes	Mashed cauliflower
Rice	Grated cauliflower
French Fries	Sliced Turnips or Zucchini
Flour	Almond or coconut flour or protein powder

Ketchup	Tomato paste, water, and stevia
Pancakes	Protein powder, eggs, and a bit of water
Cookies	Almond or coconut flour in place of flour
Ice Cream	Make your own using 35% cream, coconut milk, or almond milk or look for low-carb alternatives in store
Sorbet	Frozen fruit, coconut milk or almond milk, and stevia to taste
Pie Crust	Ground almonds
Spaghetti	Spaghetti Squash
Shepherd's Pie	Replace potatoes with mashed cauliflower
Lasagna	Replace noodles with eggplant or zucchini
Pizza	Crusts can be made out of cauliflower, zucchini, almond flour, and eggplant.

One Week Meal Plan Sample

While there is an endless supply of different variations to a low-carb meal plan one can find and learn online, it is imperative to at least start off knowing a few basic meal plan ideas to kick start your low-carb dieting efforts. I have provided some ideas for each meal category to get you started. It is important to expand your low-carb dieting meal variations. Have a look at some of the links and cookbooks provided in the resources chapter of this book for more cooking ideas.

Monday

- **Breakfast**: Omelet with bell peppers and mushrooms, fried in butter or coconut oil
- **Snack**: Sugar-free Jell-O with whipped cream
- **Lunch**: Cheeseburger (no bun), served with zucchini "fries" and salsa
- **Snack**: Pork rinds
- **Dinner**: Chicken breast, served with roasted vegetables and a small salad

Tuesday

- **Breakfast**: Bacon and eggs
- **Snack**: Pepperoni sticks
- **Lunch**: Leftover burgers and veggies from the night before
- **Snack**: String cheese
- **Dinner**: Salmon with butter and parmesan-roasted asparagus

Wednesday

- **Breakfast:** Protein shake: 2 scoops of Low-carb protein powder, 1 tsp of flax/chia seeds, 2 tsp blueberries, and coconut/almond milk or water
- **Snack:** Broccoli or cauliflower with no-sugar added full fat ranch
- **Lunch:** Shrimp salad with olive oil
- **Snack:** No crust, low carb pumpkin pie with whipped cream
- **Dinner:** Grilled chicken with bacon- and onion-fried cabbage

Thursday

- **Breakfast:** Turkey egg cups (Place slices of deli turkey in a muffin tin, crack an egg open in each one and add desired spices and cheese, bake at 350 degrees for about 10 minutes)
- **Snack:** Minimum 85% dark chocolate (check the labels to make sure the carb count is low—Lindt's has about 5 net carbs for 4 big squares)
- **Lunch:** Tuna salad with olive oil, full-fat mayonnaise, and salt and pepper
- **Snack:** Jalapeno poppers (stuff jalapenos with cream cheese and wrap them with bacon, bake at 350 degrees until bacon has reached desired crispiness)
- **Dinner:** Steak and mushrooms fried in butter and caramelized onions

Friday

- **Breakfast**: No-crust spinach and ham quiche
- **Snack**: Cucumber subs (cucumbers sliced length-wise with cream cheese and desired meat on top)
- **Lunch**: Grilled chicken wings with some raw spinach on the side
- **Snack**: "Cheese crisps" (Grated hard cheese mixed with desired spices and baked on wax paper for a few minutes until melted, let harden)
- **Dinner**: Meatballs with spaghetti squash and low carb tomato sauce

Saturday

- **Breakfast**: Protein powder pancakes: 2 eggs, 2 scoops of protein powder mixed, add just enough water to form dough, and fry like a pancake. Feel free to add in some cocoa powder or cinnamon
- **Snack**: Handful of walnuts or almonds
- **Lunch**: Pork chops with vegetables
- **Snack**: Fat bombs (Coconut oil, peanut butter, cocoa powder, butter, and artificial sweetener are melted together and frozen to make delicious ready-to-go treats!). *View this recipe online at lowcarbcoach.com*
- **Dinner**: Low-carb Shepherd's Pie: ground meat base, vegetables, cauliflower to replace the potato with butter on top

Sunday

- **Breakfast:** One-minute flax muffins (flax seed meal, baking powder, sweetener, cinnamon, egg, and a bit of oil or butter are mixed together and microwaved for a bit over a minute on high. Add desired low-carb toppings or additional flavors to spice it up!)
- **Snack:** Pizza bites (mushroom caps filled with diced pepperoni, tomato sauce, and cheese, baked until cheese is bubbly)
- **Lunch:** Bacon-wrapped chicken, served with a big salad with full-fat, no sugar added dressing
- **Snack:** Peanut butter cookies (100% natural peanut butter mixed with 1 egg and cinnamon and sweetener to taste are baked by the rounded spoonful). *View this recipe online at lowcarbcoach.com*
- **Dinner:** Slow-cooked pork tenderloin, served with mashed cauliflower drizzled with butter and complemented with garlic

Other Snack Ideas

- Handful of olives
- A few slices of cheese
- Full-fat plain yogurt with a handful of blueberries
- A hard-boiled egg or two
- Baby carrots
- Leftovers from the night before
- Protein shake

Tip: Not a fan of eggs? Awaken: 30 Egg-Free and Grain-Free Breakfasts is an e-book by Karen Sorenson of lowcarboneday.com and it is absolutely amazing!

One of the great things about low-carb eating is that you can melt cheese all over your broccoli and it's perfectly fine. It just makes your food that much more satisfying. Sauté your spinach in butter and dip your celery in gobs of blue cheese. As long as you don't stimulate insulin, your body will just burn the fat and won't store it. You won't have the insulin in your system to tell your body to store the fat.

Let's Recap

1. **Healthy Eating:** Low-Carb, High-Fat, Adequate Protein

2. **Real Food** - Meat, Poultry, Fish, Shellfish, Non-Starchy Vegetables, Low-Sugar Fruit (occasionally), Wild Foods (e.g. mushrooms), Tree Nuts (not peanuts), Sea Vegetables (e.g. kelp)

3. **Good Fats** - Butter, Lard, Coconut Oil, Palm Oil, Suet & Tallow, Chicken Fat, Unfiltered Extra Virgin Olive Oil

4. **Bad Fats** - Canola Oil, Flaxseed Oil, Peanut Oil, Corn Oil, Cottonseed Oil, Sunflower Oil, Safflower Oil, Soybean Oil, Hydrogenated Oils, Margarine, Shortening

5. **Unhealthy Eating** - Processed Foods, Grains & Brans, Sugars, Polyunsaturated Fats, High-Fructose Corn Syrup, Preservatives & Additives, Synthetic Colors & Flavors, Low-Fat or Non-Fat products, Unfermented Soy Products, Fruit Juices & Dried Fruit, Artificial Sweeteners

6. **Never:** Grains or brans, rice or potatoes, unfermented soy, industrial fats and oils, legumes or peanuts, milk, honey or agave syrup, artificial sweeteners, high sugar fruit, juices or dried fruit, starchy vegetables, processed foods, fake food sugars, high fructose corn syrup, additives or nitrates.

It seems as though when you're eating this way, you're giving up a lot, right? Remember, you're gaining more than you're giving up. Carbs give you acne, make you less able to control your weight, make you more depressed, and give you gas and heartburn. Carbs are bad for your long-term health in many ways. Every time I have slacked off and eaten carbs for a few days, my quality of life went dramatically downhill. The only thing that would improve is a pleasurable sensation on my tongue that didn't last very long.

When you find yourself concentrating on what you've lost, give equal time to what you've gained. It feels great to be slim. Take it from me, it is truly a great relief not to have to think about food all the time, which carbs tend to make you do. As a bonus, it's nice to eat the so-called "heart attack" foods, such as steak and eggs, bacon, and lobster drenched with butter, all while losing weight and feeling great.

CHAPTER FIVE

Your First Stall

So, you have been following your low-carb lifestyle to the letter but the scale doesn't move. Are you sure that you are not losing fat or better yet inches? Remember, in the Getting Started chapter, I suggested taking your measurements: now you see why.

You may not be losing weight, but is your body fat percentage going down? Are you losing inches? If you are, the weight will come with time. It's normal for your body to go through adjustment periods while you're losing weight, and not losing weight for 2-4 weeks is no cause for an alarm.

Also, have you been exercising? Muscle weighs more than fat, so if you have been building muscle, you may be losing fat but gaining muscle (weight), and that's a good thing!

Possible Causes

- <u>Too many carbs</u>: If you have started adding back carbs to your diet, perhaps the amount of carbs by which you have increased is too much for your body. Try going back to the basics and eating less than 30 carbs per day if you want to jumpstart your weight loss, or try decrementing your carb intake by 5 grams per week until you start losing weight again. Then, eat at that amount until you've reached your goal weight.

- <u>Fillers</u>: Be careful eating packaged foods or deli meat. Almost all of these products contain fillers (e.g. wheat, bran, oats, bread crumbs, and soy). Not only is this bad for people with food intolerances, it contains unnecessary carbs.

- <u>Carb Creep</u>: If you're not paying close attention, the carbs will quickly add up to an extra 10-15 carbs a day. This might not be a problem for some people, but it can stall the weight loss of those that are insulin-resistant. Try limiting the amount of salad dressings, processed meats (e.g. bacon, sausage, deli meats), and cream if you use it in your coffee/tea. If you haven't already, keep a food journal and track the number of carbohydrates and fibers you eat per day, and make sure to weigh your food (food scales can be bought inexpensively online). While eating low-carb, it's easy to lose track of how many carbs you actually eat per day, and it can have the latte effect where you think you're eating 50 net carbs, but it's actually closer to 90.

- Serving/Portion Size: When looking at packaged foods, the only thing you can trust is the nutrition label and ingredients list. If you look on the front of most packages, you can see all kinds of nice comfort words such as "sugar-free", "no added sugar", or "natural sugar", but remember that 0 carbs doesn't actually mean zero. In fact, carbs only have to be reported on the food label if there is more than 1 carb per serving in the USA or 0.5 carb per serving in Canada. This is why most food packages make the portion size small. How many people can eat ¼ cup of ice cream or 10 chips? Not me.

- Starvation: Maybe you're so used to not being able to eat from past low-fat or low-calorie diets and you're starving yourself. It's hard to understand that on a low-carb diet, you can actually eat more calories and fat and still shed those pounds. If you are not eating enough, your body will go into starvation mode and will start slowing down your metabolism and conserving energy (storing fat). Eat as much as you need until you're full. There is no need to limit the amount of protein and good fats on a low-carb diet.

- Water: Drinking enough water is even more important on a low-carb lifestyle. Water helps flush fat, aides the liver in processing protein, and removes the wastes and by-products of all that fat burning. You should be drinking at least 8 glasses of water daily, but I often drink even more.

- Medications: There are several medications that can hinder your weight loss. Diuretics, antidepressants, steroids, hormones (e.g. cortisone, birth control pills, and estrogens), as well as seizure medications. Unfortunately, any medications that you are taking to lower your cholesterol will slow the liver from burning fat and will prevent the liver from converting fat to glycogen. This is also true for diabetics taking insulin and oral diabetic medications. **Do not stop or decrease your medications without a doctor's supervision and follow-up.**

- Food Allergy or Intolerance: As you know based on the chapter My Struggle, I have been prone to several food intolerances. Many people are allergic or intolerant to soy, dairy, or gluten. Eating these foods can cause water retention, slower digestion, and a slew of other problems. If you are doing everything right, try eliminating soy, dairy, and gluten one month at a time.

Tips and Tricks

- Compare your measurements: Go back to your initial measurements and compare against your current measurements. Are you losing fat? Are you gaining muscle? Are you losing inches?

- Eat before you're hungry: If being on a low-carb diet meant that I had to have willpower, I wouldn't be on it. Always eat before you're hungry, otherwise you will have cravings, and may eat more or eat the wrong foods. Eat several small meals and snacks approximately every 3 hours.

- Don't restrict calories: If you start reducing your calories, your body will turn on "starvation mode" and start conserving your body fat instead of burning it. Eat healthy low-carb snacks such as high-fat cheese, yogurt, olives, walnuts, vegetables, fish, and eggs.

- Don't ignore the benefits of exercise: Many people are attracted to low-carb diets due to the fact that they promise to help melt the pounds without the need for exercise. While this may be true, your body will be better able to burn fat if you exercise. Additionally, those who are severely overweight may find themselves with lots of loose skin as the weight comes off. Exercise will build muscle that will keep the skin tighter.

- Avoid bedtime carbs: If you must eat something before bed, make sure it's not carbs. Have an egg, a few slices of cheese, or a handful of nuts instead.

- Remove any temptation: If you haven't already, then have a look inside your refrigerator/pantry and remove all junk foods, such as pastries, soft drinks and potato chips. Also be sure to remove all the rice, pasta, bread and grain products. This is a great opportunity to donate to your local food bank. For more tips and tricks, make sure to check out _lowcarbcoach.com_!

- Avoid cheat days: It takes up to 14 days for your body to convert from carb-burning mode to fat-burning mode. If every few days you start having a high-carb treat, you will always be stuck in the middle and never be in prime fat burning mode.

- Fat Fast: If none of the above suggestions work, try having a fat fast for three or so days where your diet consists of at least 80% fat, roughly 5% carbohydrates, and 10% protein. Try keeping your calories between 1000 and 1200 per day for these three days; this will most likely jumpstart your weight loss as in ketosis you need to eat more fat to burn more fat.

CHAPTER SIX

Common Mistakes

It is easy to make small mistakes that have a big impact throughout the journey of your low-carb diet. You need to make sure that you know all the facts before you give up on what could be the best change you make in your life!

Alcohol Intake

When consuming alcoholic beverages, your body will first burn the alcohol before going to the fat stores. This can slow down your weight loss and give you cravings. If you're going to have alcohol, have it sparingly, and choose spirits over wines or ales.

Natural Sweeteners

"Natural" sweeteners are gaining popularity to ease fears about white sugar and high-fructose corn syrup. Although it's fast becoming the preferred sweetener for health-conscious consumers, the truth is these "natural" sugars are often worse than plain table sugar.

Agave nectar, date sugar, fruit juice concentrate, honey, maple syrup, molasses, and palm/coconut sugar all break down into glucose requiring insulin. As we learned from the Low-Carb Explained chapter, anytime insulin is released, you store fat and your body stops burning fat!

Did you know that Agave nectar or syrup is as high as 90% concentrated fructose compared to the 55% fructose of high-fructose corn syrup? Don't be dazzled by words like "natural".

Sugar-Free Substitutes

While not scientifically proven, it is my opinion that for some people, the mere taste of sweet has an impact on insulin release. It's for this reason that, if you are having problems losing weight or if you are diabetic, then you should avoid or extremely limit the following.

Artificial Sweeteners – Acesulfame potassium (Sunett, Sweet One), Aspartame (Equal, NutraSweet), Saccharin (Sugar Twin, Sweet'N Low), and Sucralose (Splenda).

Sugar Alcohols – Erythritol, Hydrogenated starch Hydrolysate, Isomalt, Lactitol, Maltitol, Mannitol, Sorbitol, and Xylitol.

Novel sweeteners – Stevia extracts (Pure Via, Truvia), Tagatose (Naturlose), and Trehalose.

Are You Afraid of Eating Fat?

Most people get the majority of their calories from dietary carbohydrates, especially sugars and grains. When you remove this energy source from the diet, you must replace it with something or you will starve. Unfortunately, some people believe that because low-carb is a good idea, then low-fat AND low-carb will be even better. This is a big mistake.

You need to get energy from somewhere and if you don't eat carbs, then you MUST add in fat to compensate. If you don't, you will get hungry, feel like crap and eventually give up on the plan.

There's no scientific reason to fear fat, as long as you choose healthy fats, like saturated, monounsaturated and Omega-3s while keeping the vegetable oils to a minimum and eliminating trans-fats. For a comprehensive list of what fats to avoid, along with other foods to avoid, visit _lowcarbcoach.com_. You may be thinking that if you have to avoid foods, then what difference does this diet make from other ones that deprive you from goods? Well, the difference is that while low-carb takes certain goods away, it replaces them with other, equally tasty foods, so you'll never feel like you're at a loss!

Use of Low-Carb Packaged Foods

When buying low-carb foods that are packaged, it is of great importance to understand the ingredients. Most of these products contain soy, sugar alcohols, and even wheat. You must be very careful with these products and experiment to determine their impact on your weight loss.

Trusting the Food Packaging

Food packaging and labeling is all about marketing. When you see things like "light" or "low-carb" or "diet friendly" or "health check", you need to remember that they don't mean a thing. Read the nutritional panel; it's the one place on the entire package where they have to tell the truth!

Not Reading Food Labels

Until you get used to what is really high-carb and what isn't, make sure you check the nutritional panels of everything. Some things that you would think are low-carb really aren't (like BBQ or tomato sauce)! Some of the things you think would be high-carb aren't at all (cream, for example). Until you've been low-carbing for a while, check everything! Also, remember that food companies try and change the portion size so that it looks super low-carb. As long as the portion size has less than 0.5 carbs, they can report it as 0 carbs. Always assume that it's 0.5 carbs per serving.

Not Having a Variety of Food Available

Oftentimes, people give up on low-carb diets because of the lack of variety, although the reality is that variety shouldn't be an issue. Low-carbing means being a bit prepared, knowing what you can and can't have, and keeping foods that you can have on hand. If you let yourself get hungry and don't have quick and easy snacks, you'll end up eating the wrong things and blowing your low-carb diet.

Giving yourself cheat days

If you are breaking from your low-carb diet every few days, you will never end up in ketosis, and your body will never convert into fat-burning mode. Once you have lost your weight and have started keeping it off, it's okay to have a few indulgences.

Eating Frankenfoods

Don't eat shakes, meal bars, muffin mixes, and etcetera. Eat real food. The few times I've resorted to my emergency stash of meal bars, my weight loss suffered.

Light Salad Dressings, Dips, and Sauces

Although they are lower in calories, "light" versions of anything can be the low-carb dieter's nightmare. Why? Because anything that is light is done so by replacing the fat with carbs and/or sugar. You are better off with the full-fat versions when on a low-carb diet.

Nuts and seeds

Nuts contain a high amount of carbs. For example, 100% all natural peanut butter has 2 carbs per 1 tablespoon serving. It's way too easy to scoop out far more than you need or resort to nuts and seeds instead of protein or fat-rich foods.

CHAPTER SEVEN

Eating Out

In a perfect world, we would all be able to eat healthy home-cooked foods for every meal, but unfortunately that's not the case today. With our busy schedules, it's tough for us to always eat healthy meals from home. The key to eating out on a low-carb diet is planning.

Before going to the restaurant, you should know what you are going to eat and what you're not. What will you say to your spouse or friends when they offer you that slice of bread or a taste of their high-carb dessert? Planning ahead before you get to the restaurant will allow you to make better decisions and not be put on the spot at the restaurant.

Several restaurant chains are now offering low-carb menu options, and for those that are not, by adhering to a few basic principles, you can sample all that the world has to offer with no guilt whatsoever.

Don't Be Shy

- Restaurants are in the service business. Do not hesitate to ask for the list of ingredients that goes into a meal, entree, or sauce. Waitresses and servers are more than willing to make any changes that you wish, especially in these tough economic times.

- Tip and patronize the places that are willing to cater to your diet and substitutions. Reward your waitresses and servers for making your meal enjoyable. The opposite is also true. Some places charge more for substitutions or complain about doing it. Do not go back to these places, but before you leave, tell the manager why you will not be coming back.

- Don't be a low-carb snob. When your friends or other restaurant patrons are eating high-carb foods, don't look down on them. Remember that you were once in their shoes and that they may see your food choices and decide to change their choices in their own time.

- Plan ahead. Call the establishment and ask them about their low-carb menu options or their policy on substitutions. If the cuisine at the restaurant is typically high-carb, be sure to bring a list of acceptable foods before going. Also be sure to read the reviews for this restaurant.

- Just because something appears in the healthy section of the menu doesn't mean it is low-carb.

Basic Principles

- Salad dressings and sauces are often loaded with sugar--always ask for these on the side. This will allow you to control the amount of carbs. If you already have a favorite sauce or salad dressing, simply bring it with you. I personally use Macadamia butter.

- Stick with salad dressings that have an oil and vinegar base, such as French, Italian or Greek dressings. Mayonnaise is fine as well as Ranch dressing, which is sour cream-based.

- Replace your fries, pasta, and potatoes with vegetables or salad.

- Pass over the complimentary bread basket or chips. Advise waitress or server to not bring these out so you're not tempted.

- When possible, choose fats such as olive oil and coconut oil over industrial vegetable/seed oils or trans-fats.

- Replace the bun on your hamburger/cheeseburger with extra toppings. If you have a food allergy to gluten or eggs, be sure to ask your waitress or server, as most restaurant burgers contain binders of eggs or bread crumbs.

- Always ask for your salad to be served without croutons, and remember to have the dressing on the side.

Real Life Examples

- Buffets: You heard me right. You can go to a buffet, but be sure to stay on your diet and eat allowed low-carb foods. Avoid anything breaded or with a sauce. Most sauces generally contain sugar, cornstarch, or other non carb-friendly ingredients.

- Salad Bars or Deli: Stick to French, Italian, Ranch or Greek dressings. Mayonnaise is also okay. Avoid the bread crumbs, croutons, and highly processed vegetable oils. You can have the soup, just try and filter out the pasta or potatoes.

- Steak Houses: Avoid the bread basket and replace your baked potato with vegetables or a salad. If you're hungry, put some butter on your steak, it tastes great!

- Mongolian Grills: Pass over the soup and rice and be sure to choose low-carb vegetables. Try and stick with oil-based sauces.

- Mexican: Pass over the complimentary chips. Ask for fajitas without the beans, rice, or tortillas. Often they will give you more vegetables instead. You can also have the Chimichurri sauce. It's a thick mix of oil and greens like parsley and cilantro. Guacamole is also a great choice.

- Pub Food: Be sure to ask for naked chicken wings as most are breaded. Most pubs have burgers or steaks, which are also good choices.

- Burger Joints: Simply exchange the fries or potato for a salad or vegetables and replace the bun with extra toppings. Be careful to avoid the ketchup, it's about 2 carbs per 1 tsp!

- Chicken Places: Most chicken places now offer grilled chicken that is not breaded.

- Italian: Just have a Caesar salad without the croutons.

- Pizza: Eat the toppings and throw away the crust.

- Fast Food: Yes, you can eat at fast food places and still eat low-carb. KFC offers grilled chicken *breast that's not breaded. Carl's Jr offers a low-carb burger, and at places like Harvey's, McDonald's, Burger King, and Wendy's, you can simply ask for it on a plate with no bun.

- Japanese: You'll want to avoid eating sushi because of the white rice, but sashimi offers the same wonderful flavors.

CHAPTER EIGHT

Myths

There are a number of myths regarding the weight loss as well as other aspects of the low-carb diet program.

The truth behind these will be different. These are generally followed by the people who like to lose their weight or are trying to manage their diabetes. Exercising is also very important for maintaining the body, but following some restricted diet helps just the same with reaching your goal weight while keeping your body healthy. As these low-carb diets cause more weight loss, and even minimize several risk factors for a disease, following them is always safe if used correctly, and provided you don't have a history of liver failure.

Is Most of the Weight Lost Water?

A portion of the initial weight loss is water, just as it is on any diet. It takes about 4 days of reducing your carbs to less than 20-30 grams of carbs per day before your body changes to burning fat.

Will Eating More Protein Lead to Kidney Damage?

There has never been a study that demonstrated increasing protein intake damages healthy kidneys. However, people who already have severe pre-existing kidney disease often require a more limited protein intake along with regular monitoring of kidney function.

People with diabetes are at risk for kidney disease. Not because of eating protein, but because of the damaging effects of high levels of blood sugar. Controlling carbohydrates is a good strategy for improving blood sugar control in people with type II diabetes; therefore, decreasing the risk of kidney complications as well as other complications of diabetes.

Doesn't a Low-Carb Diet Cause Osteoporosis?

A number of studies have shown the importance of adequate protein for bone health. The Framingham Osteoporosis Study demonstrated the importance of dietary protein for building and maintaining strong bones especially as one ages. Over a four-year period, the elderly people who ate the most protein had the strongest bones. Those who ate the least lost significantly more bone mass. Now just imagine what a youthful state you'd be in while in your old age if you combined your low-carb diet with strength training! You can imagine it as a gift to your future self, rather than constantly thinking that you need things "now".

Doesn't a High-Fat Diet Cause Cancer?

Consuming natural fats do not lead to cancer. Having a high body fat percentage predisposes you to cancer. Fat is often blamed, because fat is higher in calories than protein or carbo-hydrates, and the assumption is made that eating higher fat will make you fat, based on the calories-in-calories-out theory. When following a low-carb lifestyle, you are not gaining fat but burning it and normalizing your weight.

Won't Low-Carb Diets Cause Liver Damage?

There has never been any research to support this. It is likely another theory that because low-carb dieters consume a higher fat intake it will cause fatty infiltration of the liver. All of the studies done on people following Atkins have examined liver function tests on previously healthy livers and have shown it to be safe.

Isn't Low-carb Just for Short-Term Weight Loss?

Low-carb diets have been around since 1860 and should be called a "lifestyle" and not diet. To be successful in managing weight, you must make permanent changes in what you eat and how you make your food decisions.

Don't High-Fat Diets Cause Heart Disease?

The idea that dietary cholesterol and saturated fat leads to heart disease is only a theory. For an eye-opening and interesting dis-cussion on how this theory came to be adopted, read *Good Calories, Bad Calories* by Gary Taubes.

Low-carb diets decrease cardiovascular risks by:

- Re-balancing blood sugar/insulin
- Lowering triglycerides
- Increasing HDL cholesterol better than any drug available

- Shifting LDL particles from small, dangerous types to large, buoyant particles
- Decreasing inflammatory chemicals
- Lowering blood pressure, decreasing fluid retention
- Improving the processing of saturated fat
- Inhibiting the manufacturing of fat
- Improving the clearance/use of saturated fat

But Doesn't Your Body Need Carbs?

Unlike fat and protein, there is no minimum daily dietary need for carbs, although you will hear this statement made all the time. Yes, the brain and few other tissues in the body require about 130 grams of carbs daily to function properly, but these need not be from food sources. The body is quite capable of meeting this need by making enough glucose for these tissues. Additionally, the brain and heart function efficiently on ketones. If our bodies couldn't do this, our species would not have survived. Ketones are produced when fat is burned, which happens when you cut carbs to less than 50 grams daily. Remember that your fat reserves are there as fuel stores to prevent starvation and protect lean mass. If you have an excess of fat stores, what better way to use them than for fuel, as they were intended?

Wouldn't You Always Be Tired?

Quite the contrary; controlling both the quality and quantity of carbs stabilizes blood sugar and insulin levels, leading to more energy and more sustained energy. It can take a few days for the body to adapt to a fat-burning metabolism rather than a glucose-burning one. During that time, some people may experience fatigue. Additionally, because high insulin levels cause water retention, as high levels normalize, fatigue can occur if too much water is lost and with it minerals. To avoid this, have two cups of hot water with salty bouillon along with your lunch daily, or take a multi-mineral containing calcium, potassium and magnesium.

Sugar gives you very short-term energy, and in many people actually causes a hypoglycemic response leading to fatigue and numerous other symptoms within two hours or so of your last sugar fix.

Research has demonstrated that fat burning provides more sustained energy once you have adapted to a fat-burning metabolism. This has been tested on competitive athletes whose energy requirements are far above the average person's.

Don't Doctors Promote Low-Fat Diets?

Modern society has largely been indoctrinated into the mindset that fat clogs your arteries and makes you fat, and should thus be avoided. But nothing could be further from the truth. Tropical oils, like coconut and palm, as well as butter from grass-fed animals and fat derived from meat are actually quite healthy for you. These saturated fats help promote healthy brain function and regulate proper hormone production. Popular vegetable oils, on the other hand, which oftentimes are hydrogenated and morphed into trans-fats, are a primary cause of heart disease and other illness, and should be avoided.

Shouldn't We Be Eating Less Salt?

This claim assumes that most people are consuming high amounts of synthetic, refined table salt, which is highly toxic and responsible for causing widespread cellular inflammation, hence the many warnings about salt intake. But what most people do not know is that unrefined, all-natural sea salt and mineral salts are completely different, as they are packed with health-promoting minerals, electrolytes, and other important nutrients. Eating lots of sea and mineral salt, in other words, is actually good for your health.

Isn't Natural Sugar Good For You?

In most cases, switching out that table sugar for honey or agave nectar in the name of improving health is a misnomer, as these popular sugar substitutes are sometimes just as refined and unhealthy as regular sugar. Agave, for instance, contains high levels of fructose, which is metabolized directly by the liver and turned into fat. And unless your honey is raw, unprocessed, and locally sourced, it is also a toxic offender when consumed liberally.

Don't Eggs Raise Your Cholesterol?

The medical system has gone back-and-forth on this one, but the truth about eggs will always remain the same: pasture-raised eggs from healthy chickens are an excellent source of both protein and cholesterol, and they are not in and of themselves a cause of heart disease. And removing egg yolks and eating only the whites, as many people now do, can actually be detrimental to your health, as eggs should be eaten in complete form for optimal nutrition.

Isn't Red Meat Unhealthy?

The mainstream media loves to target red meat these days, but the problem with telling people to limit their consumption of red meat in order to avoid heart disease is that not all red meat is the same. In fact, red meat from grass-fed, pasture-raised cattle is actually just as healthy as, and potentially even healthier than, wild-caught salmon. This contrasts sharply with factory-farmed red meat which is high in pro-inflammatory Omega-6 fatty acids. It is all about how the animals are raised and what they are eating that determines the nutritional profile of meat in general, which is why it is always best to choose meat from local, naturally-raised sources.

Doesn't Low-Carb Mean No-Carb?

While it may feel like it at first, following a low-carb way of eating does not mean that you do not eat any carbs. While some plans have greater allowances than others, it all comes down to the individual. As with anything in life, you learn where you feel and function best. The average American consumes 300 grams of carbs per day, if not more. (It's usually way more.) Most low-carb plans will put you at a level under 100 grams of carbs per day. For me, I feel my best when I eat under 40 grams a day. Again, these are net carbs; visit _lowcarbcoach.com_ for more examples on the difference between net carbs versus carbs.

I Heard You Don't Eat Fruit or Vegetables?

Quite the opposite! While on a low-carb way of eating, this is where the majority of your carbs come from. Starchy vegetables (like white potato, peas, and carrots) and high sugar fruits (like pineapple, bananas, and grapes) are not encouraged, but non-starchy vegetables and low-sugar fruits (like raspberries) are.

Won't You Have Heart Disease or High Cholesterol?

Again, the opposite; study after study has shown that people on a low-carbohydrate diet LOWER their risk for heart disease, and their cholesterol actually improves. You'll be seeing me add a section where news articles, medical studies, and other low-carb scientific data are complied. I'm sure you'll find this information very interesting!

Don't People On Low-Carb Diets Lose Muscle?

Not true. In fact, low-carb diets are better at preserving and even increasing lean muscle mass. In a study published in 1984, a team of scientists from MIT and Harvard studied two groups of overweight women. They put one group on a low-carb diet, and the other group on a high-carb diet. Each diet allowed 700 calories per day. Even with a severe caloric deficit, the greater percentage of protein consumed on the low-carb diet and the effects of ketosis resulted in a greater retention of muscle mass for the subjects on the low-carb diet. In other words, the subjects on the high-carb diet lost more muscle mass because the carbs they were eating displaced some of the protein that would have helped them retain muscle mass.

This phenomenon of how dietary protein helps the body retain muscle mass has been shown many times over in various studies on very-low-calorie diets, which include adequate protein and muscle building substrates, such as sodium and potassium.

This general "muscle wasting" assertion often comes from trainers and dietitians who really have not studied the science on muscle preservation. They will tell you that the brain requires at least 100 grams of carb per day and that if you don't get those carbs in the diet, your body will break down your muscles to get it. This is true when one's diet is high-carb, and no ketone bodies are available as an alternative source of brain fuel, but not for a person who has adapted to a low-carb, keto-genic diet. Ketosis provides fuel in the form of ketone bodies for the brain, and the requirement for glucose drops to only about 40 grams per day. The body can easily make this amount from dietary protein and glycerol from the breakdown of fatty acids.

CHAPTER NINE

Healthy Cheating

We've all had rainy days where we want to grab the nearest box of biscuits or package of Reese's and indulge like there's no tomorrow. There's no shame in it, only learning from it and discovering how to reach over for something a little smarter. Celery with peanut butter might not be the greatest thing in the world when you're craving something sweet, so I've compiled a few recipes, some from the One Week Sample Menu and some exclusive recipes, for you to enjoy! For many more recipes, pictures, and tips and tricks on these recipes (and others) go to _lowcarbcoach.com_. The beauty of these recipes is that while it might feel like you're "cheating", you're actually not as recipes are very low in carbohydrates. Naturally, this is in moderation—if you choose to eat over 50 fat bombs in one sitting then you may kick yourself out of ketosis! (I don't know if you'd want to eat that many at once, though.)

Low-Carb Peanut Butter Cookies

<u>Ingredients</u>

1 cup 100% natural peanut butter
1 teaspoon liquid stevia or equivalent
1 teaspoon baking soda
1 egg
1 teaspoon vanilla extract
1 teaspoon cinnamon

<u>Instructions</u>

1. Preheat oven to 350 degrees Fahrenheit.
2. Mix together and put a heaping teaspoon onto greased wax paper.
3. Press them down so they're cookie shaped and bake for 8-10 minutes (8 if you want them softer).

Low-Carb Almond Cookies

<u>Ingredients</u>

2 Cups of Almond Flour
2 Teaspoons of Stevia
1/2 Teaspoon of Salt
1/2 Cup Softened Unsalted Butter
1 Teaspoon Vanilla Extract
1 Egg

<u>Instructions</u>

1. Preheat the oven to 300 degrees Fahrenheit.
2. Using an electric mixer, blend the softened butter for one minute.
3. Add the remaining ingredients.
4. Form dough into walnut-sized balls and place onto ungreased cookie sheet.
5. Bake for 5 minutes. Press down lightly with a fork, and then continue to bake another 18 minutes.
6. Let cool on cookie sheet for 5 minutes before removing.

Chocolate Fat Bombs

<u>Ingredients</u>

3/4 Cup Coconut Oil (melted)
1/2 Cup Almond Butter (melted)
1/4 Teaspoon of Stevia (liquid or powdered)
3 Tablespoon Coco Powder (unsweetened)
1/2 Cup Salted Butter (melted)

<u>Instructions</u>

1. Put all the ingredients into a bowl and mix well until all the ingredients are combined.
2. Place a Silicone Brownie Bites Pan (Michaels Arts & Crafts) on top of a cookie sheet.
3. Pour 2 tablespoons of the mixture into each of the 24 molds.
4. Freeze for 30 minutes and enjoy!

CHAPTER TEN

Resources

Education is the key to having all the tools you need to make your low-carb lifestyle change successful and permanent rather than another on-again-off-again diet failure. There is no single tool that can provide all you need to know about low-carb diets. Take advantage of the following low-carb resources as well as our website *lowcarbcoach.com*.

Books

- **Good Calories, Bad Calories**: *Fats, Carbs, and the Controversial Science of Diet and Health*

- **Why We Get Fat**: *And What to Do About It*

- **Trick and Treat**: *How 'healthy eating' is making us ill*

- **New Atkins for a New You**: *The Ultimate Diet for Shedding Weight and Feeling Great*

- **Atkins Diabetes Revolution**: *The Groundbreaking Approach to Preventing and Controlling Type 2 Diabetes*

- **Dr. Atkins' Vita-Nutrient Solution**: *Nature's Answer to Drugs*

- **The Art and Science of Low-carbohydrate Performance**

- **Life Without Bread**: *How a Low-Carbohydrate Diet Can Save Your Life*

- **Know Your Fats**: *The Complete Primer for Understanding the Nutrition of Fats, Oils, and Cholesterol*

- **The Vegetarian Myth**: *Food Justice and Sustainability*

- **Cholesterol Clarity**: *What The HDL Is Wrong With My Numbers?*

Websites

- **Gary Taubes**
  http://garytaubes.com/

- **Peter Attia**
  http://eatingacademy.com/

- **Jimmy Moore**

  http://livinlavidalowcarb.com/blog/

- **NuSI**

  http://nusi.org/

- **Atkins**

  http://atkins.com/

- **Robb Wolf**

  http://robbwolf.com/

- **Mark's Daily Apple**

  http://www.marksdailyapple.com

- **Low-carb Coach**

  http://lowcarbcoach.com

- **Low-carb Canada**

  http://lowcarbcanada.ca

- **Low-carb Grocery**

  http://thelowcarbgrocery.com/

- **Jacqueline Eberstein**

  http://www.controlcarb.com/

Recipes

- **Low-carb Luxury**

  http://lowcarbluxury.com/lowcarb-recipes.html

- **Linda's Low-carb Menus & Recipes**

  http://www.genaw.com/lowcarb/recipes.html

- **Low-Carbing Among Friends**

  http://amongfriends.us/

- **Food Network**

  http://www.food.com/recipe-finder/all/low-carb

- **George Stella**

  http://stellastyle.com/site/recipes/

- **All Day I DREAM About Food**

  http://alldayidreamaboutfood.com/

- **DJ Foodie**

  http://djfoodie.com/

- **Your Lighter Side**

  http://yourlighterside.com/

- **The LowCarbist**

  http://lowcarbist.com/

CHAPTER ELEVEN

What Now?

'm sure at this point if you haven't already started your low-carb journey, you're anxious to begin. The first thing I urge you to do is to take your measurements, weigh yourself, and get a check-up to find out your vitals. Either before or after you clear out your pantry and go shopping for your new and delicious food, head on over to *lowcarbcoach.com* and join a community of other friendly low-carbers eager to help you succeed!

Every choice you make will create a small, but impactful, difference in your life in the long run—only you can decide how positive that difference will be, but we can certainly help you achieve those small differences!